THE OPTIMAL K
DISEASE COOKBOOK FOR
SENIORS

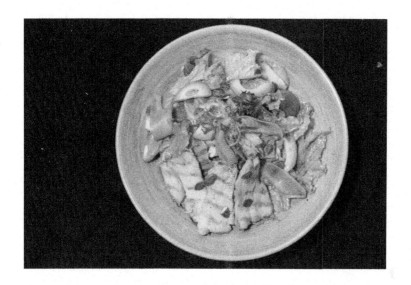

Nourishing Recipes for Managing Kidney Disease in Later Life

Presley Butler

Table of Contents

Chapter 8: Dinner 75

Chapter 9: Snacks And Desserts 97

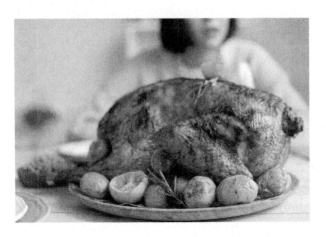

Introduction

James Frank, 62, had a kidney illness, which had been identified. He was resolved to live as long as he could in good health and kidney function. James found a renal illness diet cookbook for seniors after doing some research. It was created to help people with kidney disease improve their general health.

James was given the knowledge he needed to both maintain and improve his kidney health through the renal disease diet cookbook for seniors. He was instructed by the recipes and meal plans to reduce his intake of sodium, limit certain proteins and cholesterol, and eat adequate potassium and phosphorus. James was happy to learn that the cookbook offered suggestions for substitutions that would allow him to personalize and improve his meals.

The kidney disease diet cookbook for seniors initially seemed a little intimidating to James. In addition to adjusting to a new diet, he also had to learn how to cook and prepare new, healthier dishes.He made the decision to gradually add a few new recipes each week until he was at ease with his new dinner strategy.

James quickly became an expert cook thanks to some useful advice from the kidney disease diet cookbook for seniors and some trial and error. Unexpectedly, he discovered that he was loving the task and the gratification of making a dinner that was delicious and considerate of his kidney function.

James eventually experienced an uptick in energy, a decrease in weariness, and an overall improvement in his health as the weeks passed. In addition to assisting him in achieving the ideal mix of protein, potassium, and acid-base intake, his meals also gave him access to healthy dietary fiber and vital vitamins.

As our society ages, the nutritional requirements of seniors with kidney disease become more and more significant. Seniors with this condition must follow a diet that is well-balanced and supportive of their kidneys. This cookbook provides a selection of dishes created especially to satisfy the dietary requirements of people with kidney disease while also preserving the pleasure and satisfaction that comes from eating delectable meals. This cookbook is filled with delicious, nutrient-dense selections that will please the palates of elderly citizens with kidney disease, from quick and simple appetizers to robust main dishes to guilt-free sweets. This cookbook offers seniors with kidney disease the chance to maintain their health and partake in delectable food, thanks to its simple explanations of how to incorporate renal disease diet-friendly components into meals.

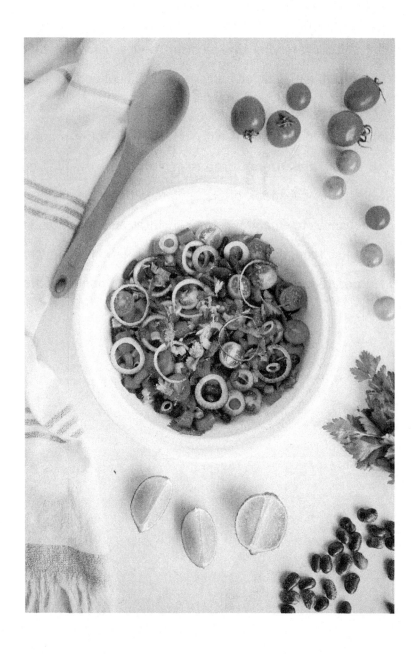

Chapter 1: Fundamentals and Types of Kidney Disease

Nephropathy, commonly referred to as renal disease or kidney disease, is a medical disorder in which the kidneys' capacity to generate urine and filter toxins from the blood is compromised. Since kidney disease is a progressive condition, it deteriorates over time. As the condition worsens, symptoms like nausea, vomiting, weight loss, exhaustion, swelling in the legs and ankles, and difficulties concentrating may also appear. The most severe stage of kidney illness, end-stage renal disease (ESRD), necessitates dialysis or a kidney transplant for treatment.

Structure, function, and clinical implications are the three primary divisions of the foundations of kidney disease. The abdominal cavity contains two bean-shaped organs called kidneys, one on both sides of the spine. A network of capillaries and glomeruli, which are specialized capillaries that remove toxins from the blood, make up each kidney's individual filtration system. The collecting ducts, which are in charge of making and transporting urine, are also housed within the kidneys. The kidneys' job is to filter blood, get rid of poisons from it, and make urine. The kidneys also create hormones necessary for the creation of red blood cells and control the body's salt, potassium, and acid-base balances.

The underlying cause and severity of kidney disease determine its clinical effects. While some people's kidney function may gradually but noticeably diminish, others may experience an abrupt, quick decline. Patients may report weariness, trouble focusing, and changes in urine, such as more frequent urination or nocturnal urination, in either scenario. High blood pressure and diabetic complications are the two most common causes of renal damage which may be managed with dietary adjustments, physical activity, and weight reduction. The chance of getting kidney disease can also be increased by other lifestyle choices, such as smoking.

1. Acute kidney injury (AKI), also known as acute kidney failure, can have a variety of reasons, such as dehydration,

drugs, or infections. It develops suddenly over a few days or weeks. Medication, fluids, and bed rest are frequently used as treatments.

2. Chronic kidney disease (CKD): This form of kidney disease develops slowly over many years and is typically brought on by diabetes or high blood pressure. Complications include anemia, bone disease, and heart disease might result from it. Treatment typically involves making lifestyle changes, taking drugs, and having the underlying ailment treated through procedures.

3. Polycystic kidney disease (PKD): This form of kidney disease is an inherited illness that damages and impairs kidney function by causing cysts to grow inside the organs. Medication and food changes are frequently part of treatment.

4. Glomerular disease: The kidney's glomeruli, or small filters, are affected by this type of kidney disease. It can result in renal impairment and is frequently brought on by autoimmune diseases or infections. Medication, dietary

changes, and routine kidney function monitoring are common treatment options.

5. Hypertensive Nephropathy: High blood pressure affects the tiny blood arteries in the kidney, resulting in this type of kidney disease. Medication, dietary changes, and ongoing kidney function monitoring are common treatment options.

6. Interstitial nephritis: The tissues encircling the kidneys' filtering organs become inflamed in this form of kidney disease. It might appear out of the blue or accompany a urinary tract infection. Medication, antibiotics, and renal function monitoring are frequently used as treatments.

7. Nephrotic syndrome: This kidney disease is brought on by protein loss through the urine and may have a number of underlying causes. Medication is frequently used as part of treatment to lower urine protein levels and enhance child

Chapter 2: Do's and Don'ts while on Kidney Disease Diet:

Do's

1. To acquire the vitamins and minerals that support kidney function, consume a lot of fresh fruits and vegetables.

2. Sip on a lot of liquids; daily goal should be somewhere between eight and ten glasses of water.

3. Keep an eye out for meals strong in potassium-rich vitamins, minerals, and other nutrients, and monitor your potassium intake.

4. Consume modest amounts of protein to aid the kidneys in their filtering work.

5. Opt for complex carbs such as whole grains and whole wheat bread over simple carbohydrates like those found in processed foods.

6. Consume low-sodium foods to aid in lowering blood pressure and fluid retention.

7. To assist prevent further kidney issues, speak with your doctor or nutritionist about other specific dietary modifications.

Don'ts:

1. Refrain from consuming sugary foods and beverages because they can harm your kidneys.

2. Limit your protein intake, as the kidneys must work harder to process it.

3. Avoid salt, which makes you retain more fluid.

4. Stay clear of foods and drinks high in phosphorus, such as dairy goods, red meat, nuts, whole grain breads, bean products, and some sodas.

5. Resist drinking because it interferes with the kidney's capacity to filter toxins.

6. Steer clear of processed foods, which are frequently heavy in sugar, salt, and other potentially dangerous ingredients.

7. Discuss any extra dietary limitations you might need to adhere to with your doctor.

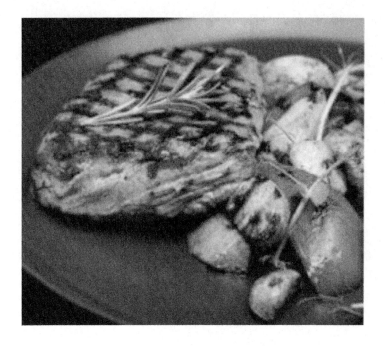

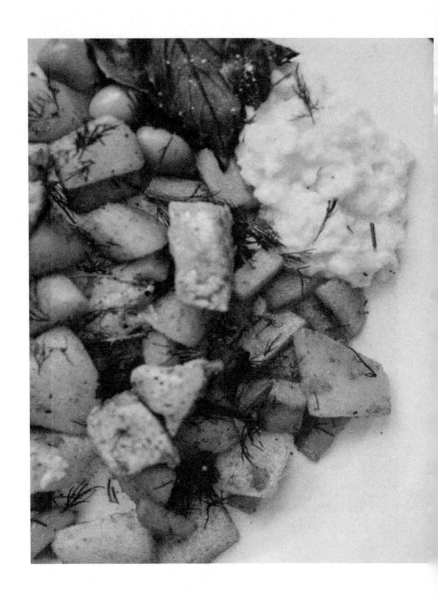

Chapter 3: Meal Planning and Portion Control

A geriatric diet for kidney disease should include meal planning and portion control. Eating the correct meals in the proper proportions can lower the risk of significant health issues while maintaining renal health. A kidney-friendly meal plan should include a range of nutrient- and fiber-rich foods, like whole grains, low-fat dairy products, lean proteins, and fruits and veggies, to maintain optimal nutrition and health.

Planning meals requires keeping an eye on the size of the servings. Consuming too much food can strain the kidneys and raise one's risk of type 2 diabetes, high blood pressure, and other diseases. Eating out or in a restaurant can also be difficult because the portions are frequently larger than necessary. Limiting servings of proteins to 3–4 ounces, carbohydrates to 1–2 cups, and vegetables to 1–cup is a useful approach for managing portion sizes.

Another crucial component of a kidney-friendly diet is fluid intake. An accumulation of substances in the bloodstream brought on by excessive fluid intake might harm the kidneys. Seniors should keep their daily fluid intake to no more than 8 cups to reduce this risk.

There may be additional dietary limitations that must be followed for people who have renal insufficiency. Examples include reducing potassium and phosphorus intake, avoiding nuts and legumes, and avoiding foods high in sodium. The ideal diet for a certain patient can be determined with the advice of a nutritionist or medical professional.

Chapter 4: Examining Nutrition Labels to Avoid Substances That Could Damage Your Kidneys

If you're following a renal disease diet, it's crucial that you carefully read food labels. You may choose nutritious foods and improve your condition by being aware of what is in the food you eat.

Look for Total calories, fat, cholesterol, salt, carbohydrates, and protein in the nutritional profile on the label. The best strategy to maintain a healthy renal diet is to consume meals that are low in sodium, cholesterol, and fat and contain sufficient levels of protein and natural carbohydrates.

A diet for kidney illness should include reading food labels. By learning what the labels mean, You can rest assured that you are eating the appropriate things and avoiding substances that could damage your kidneys.

The nutrition data should be your first stop when reading a food label. You may find out in this section how much salt, cholesterol, sugar, protein, fat, and carbs are in each serving. While eating foods high in fat, carbohydrates, sugar, and sodium can be hazardous, eating foods higher in protein can assist maintain renal function.

The list of ingredients is the next crucial item to check. Avoid eating items that may damage your kidneys because they include additives, preservatives, or flavors. Foods high in phosphorus should be avoided since they might be stressful for your kidneys. Red meat, dairy products, processed foods, and soda are a few typical sources of high-phosphorus diets.

Finally, scan the label's end for allergies. Avoid the product or take the required safety in the event that it includes any allergens to which you are allergic; precautions will be taken to guarantee that it is safe for ingestion.

Following these suggestions and carefully reading food labels can make it simpler to ensure you are receiving the right amount of nutrients from each item. The nutritional values should be changed to reflect the bigger portion size if you frequently consume more than the serving size.

When shopping for foods that are kidney-friendly, the majority of labels will contain a brief statement that indicates if the product has any specific components, like lower salt or potassium, that can improve your kidney health. To fully comprehend the product you are eating, be careful to read the ingredients list.

It's also crucial to remember that many processed and packaged meals are high in sodium, so try to stay away from them whenever you can. The ideal foods for a kidney disease diet include fresh produce, lean meats, and fruits and vegetables.

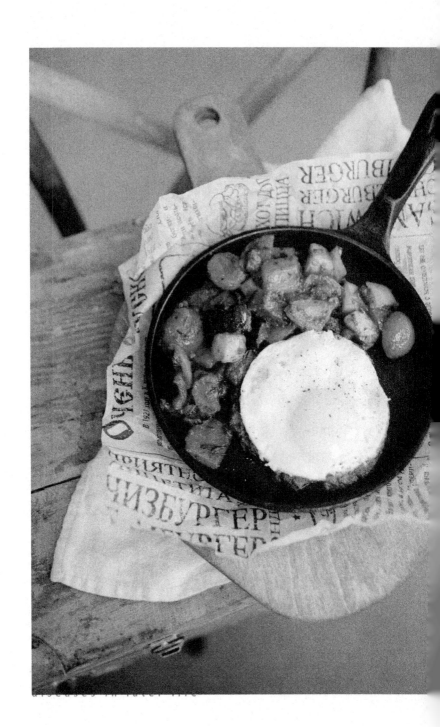

Chapter 5: Basic Nutrition for Seniors With Kidney Disease

Seniors with kidney illness should focus primarily on eating a balanced and healthy diet. Poor nutrition, which results in insufficient or inappropriate nutritional consumption, can exacerbate renal disease and cause other health problems.

Seniors with kidney illness need to be aware of their nutritional requirements. In order to maintain optimum health, some nutrients may need to be restricted. A nutritionist can collaborate with the senior to create a personalized food plan catered to their unique requirements.

Seniors with kidney disease should reduce their intake of salt, phosphorus, and potassium to maintain healthy kidney function. The water balance may be impacted by high salt levels, which are present in processed foods, and blood pressure might rise as a result. To assist preserve bone health and manage calcium levels, phosphorus intake should be kept to a minimum since it is present in dairy products, processed foods, and canned beverages. To control blood pressure, potassium intake—which is present in fruits and vegetables—should also be restricted.

Any diet should include protein, but seniors with kidney disease need it more than anyone else. Protein helps to keep muscles strong and fight weariness. Aim for 50–75g of protein per day from healthy sources such as lean meats, fish, eggs, lentils, and peas for seniors with kidney disease.

Seniors with kidney illness should drink plenty of water as well. Drinking enough water supports digestion, prevents dehydration, and assists the kidneys in removing waste. Seniors can maintain a nutritious diet by adhering to a meal plan that includes fruits and vegetables, complete grains, and lean proteins.

If seniors with renal disease pay attention to the fundamentals of diet, they may retain their wellness and standard of life. They can control their renal illness and stay healthy by eating a balanced, healthful diet and adhering to customized meal plans.

Chapter 6: Breakfast Recipes

Breakfast Burrito

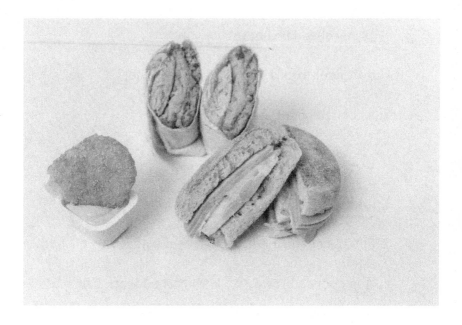

Enjoy this delicious breakfast burrito to get your day started! Due to its abundance of nutritious ingredients, it's a great way to commence the day.

Ingredients:

- 1/4 cup mashed black beans

- 1/4 cup cooked brown rice

- 1/4 cup sautéed vegetables (onions, peppers, mushrooms)

- 2 eggs

- 1/4 cup cheddar cheese

- 1 soft flour tortilla

- Salt and pepper to taste

Cooking Method:

1. Put a skillet on medium-high heat with a little oil in it.

2. Add cooked brown rice and mashed black beans to the skillet and stir to incorporate.

3. Include the sautéed vegetables and stir continuously.

4. Scramble the eggs in the skillet until they are fully done.

5. After turning off the heat, add the cheddar cheese shredded.

6. Place a flour tortilla on a dish and fill the center with the egg and bean mixture.

7. To form a burrito, fold the tortilla's sides over the filling.

To serve, divide the burrito in half.

Nutritional Value: Per serving (1 burrito)

Calories: 373

Fat: 16 g

Protein: 20 g

Carbohydrates: 35 g

Fiber: 6 g

Sugars: 3 g

Banana Oatmeal Pancakes

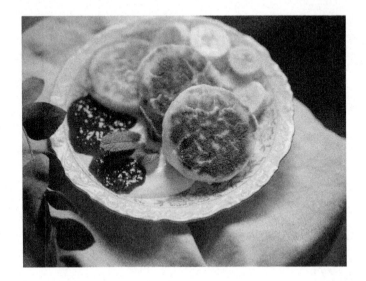

A delightful way to start your morning is with these banana oatmeal pancakes. They have a great flavor and are fluffy and airy.

Ingredients:

- 1 banana, mashed

- 1 cup quick-cooking oats

- 1/2 teaspoon baking powder

- 2 eggs

- 1/4 cup almond milk

- Pinch of ground cinnamon

- Coconut oil for cooking

Cooking Method:

1. Mash the banana in a big bowl until it's smooth.

2. Include the almond milk, cinnamon, baking soda, oats, and baking powder. Stir the ingredients together thoroughly.

3. Set a skillet that has been lightly oiled to medium heat.

4. Pour a quarter cup of the pancake batter onto the heating skillet.

5. Cook for an additional 2 minutes after flipping or until the edges begin to look dry.

6. Carry out step 6 with the remaining batter.

7. Present with your preferred garnishes.

Nutritional Value: Per serving (2 pancakes)

Calories: 157

Fat: 5 g

Protein: 7 g

Carbohydrates: 20 g

Fiber: 3 g

Sugars: 5 g

Huevos Rancheros

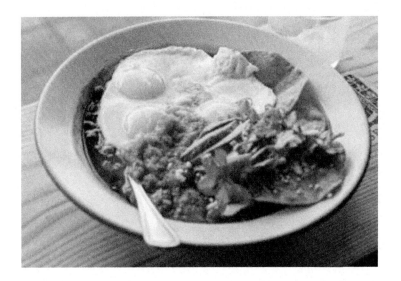

This Huevos Rancheros will make your morning brighter! As it is brimming with delicious flavors, it is an excellent way to start an exception day.

Ingredients:

- 1 tablespoon olive oil

- 1/4 cup diced onion

- 1/4 cup diced red pepper

- 1/2 teaspoon chili powder

- 2 eggs

- 2 whole-grain tortillas

- 1/4 cup black beans

- 1/4 cup salsa

- 1/4 cup cheddar cheese

- Fresh cilantro for garnish

- Salt and pepper to taste

Cooking Method:

1. In a big skillet over medium-high heat, warm the olive oil.

2. Cook the red pepper, onions, and other ingredients in the skillet for about four minutes or until tender.

3. Include the chili powder and cook for an additional minute.

4. After adding the eggs,fry for about two minutes in the skillet, depending on the desired quality.

5. Arrange the tortillas on a serving tray and top each with cheddar cheese, salsa, black beans, and eggs.

6. Add salt and pepper and garnish with fresh cilantro.

7. Serve right away.

Nutritional Value: Per serving (1 burrito)

Calories: 373

Fat: 16 g

Protein: 20 g

Carbohydrates: 35 g

Fiber: 6 g

Sugars: 3 g

Overnight Coconut Chia Oats

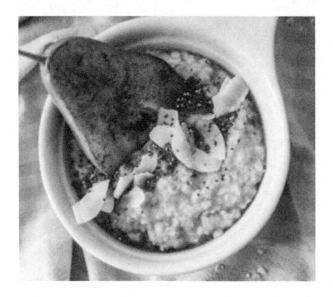

These Overnight Coconut Chia Oats are a quick and filling breakfast option. It's a superb way of kicking off the day and ready in a flash!

Ingredients:

- 1/2 cup rolled oats

- 1/2 cup shredded coconut

- 2 tablespoons chia seeds

- Pinch of ground cinnamon

- 1/2 cup almond milk

- 1/4 cup diced mango

- 2 tablespoons diced almonds

- 2 tablespoons honey (optional)

Cooking Method:

1. Combine the oats, coconut shreds, chia seeds, and cinnamon in a big bowl.

2. After adding the almond milk, whisk everything together.

3. Put the bowl's lid on and put the mixture in the refrigerator for the night.

4. Add the diced mango and almonds the following morning.

5. If desired, incorporate the honey; stir.

6. Present warm or cold.

Nutritional Value: Per serving (1 bowl)

Calories: 318

Fat: 16 g

Protein: 9 g

Carbohydrates: 33 g

Fibre: 7 g

Sugars: 11 g

Oatmeal Toast with Fruit

This oatmeal toast with fruit will make breakfast simple. This breakfast is wholesome and light thanks to a few straightforward

Ingredients:

- 1 slice whole-grain toast

- 2 tablespoons rolled oats

- 1/4 teaspoon ground cinnamon

- 1/4 cup diced fresh fruit (strawberries, blueberries, etc.)

- 2 tablespoons plain yogurt

- 1 tablespoon honey

Cooking Method:

1. Toast the piece of bread.

2. Mix the oats and cinnamon.

3. Place the oat mixture on top of the toast.

4. Top with yogurt, yogurt mixed with diced fruit and honey.

5. Enjoy!

Nutritional Value: Per serving (1 toast)

Calories: 178

Fat: 3 g

Protein: 5 g

Carbohydrates: 33 g

Fiber: 5 g

Sugars: 14 g

Chocolate Peanut Butter Overnight Oatmeal

Chocolate and peanut butter are a traditional pairing, and this breakfast dish is sure to please.

Ingredients:

- 1 cup rolled oats

- 1/2 cup unsweetened almond milk

- 2 tablespoons chia seeds

- 2 tablespoons peanut butter

- 2 tablespoons cocoa powder

- 2 tablespoons honey

- 1/4 teaspoon ground cinnamon

- 1/4 cup diced banana

Cooking Method:

1. In a big bowl, combine the oats, almond milk, chia seeds, peanut butter, chocolate powder, honey, and cinnamon.

2. Stir everything together.

3. Cover the bowl and store it overnight in the refrigerator.

4. The following morning, add the diced banana.

5. Whether cooled or at room temperature, serve

Nutritional Value: Per serving (1 serving)

Calories: 281

Fat: 10 g

Protein: 9 g

Carbohydrates: 41 g

Fiber: 6 g

Sugars: 16 g

Banana Almond French Toast

This Banana Almond French Toast will give you a delightful start to the day. It's the ideal morning start, lightly sweetened with honey and almond essence.

Ingredients:

- 2 eggs

- 2 tablespoons almond milk

- 1/2 teaspoon almond extract

- 2 slices whole grain bread

- 1 banana, thinly sliced

- 1 tablespoon honey

- 2 tablespoons sliced almonds for garnish

Cooking Method:

1. Mix the eggs, almond milk, and almond essence.

2. Dip the bread pieces into the egg mixture to coat both sides.

3. Heat a lightly oiled skillet over medium heat.

4. Place the bread cubes in the skillet and cook for two to 3 minutes or until they start to become golden. After flipping, cook for a further two minutes.

5. Spread honey over the toast and top with banana slices and nuts.

6. Serve immediately.

Nutritional Value: Per serving (1 serving)

Calories: 274

Fat: 11 g

Protein: 11 g

Carbohydrates: 34 g

Fiber: 5 g

Sugars: 18 g

Apple-Cinnamon Muffins

These apple-cinnamon muffins will fulfill your sweet tooth in the morning. They are sweet and juicy, which makes them the perfect morning pick-me-up.

Ingredients:

- 1 cup almond flour

- 1/2 cup oat flour

- 1 teaspoon baking powder

- 1/4 teaspoon ground cinnamon

- 1/4 cup brown sugar

- 2 eggs

- 1/4 cup melted coconut oil

- 1/2 cup diced apples

- 2 tablespoons chopped walnuts

- 2 tablespoons honey

Cooking Method:

1. Turn the oven's temperature to 350.

2. In a large basin, mix the brown sugar, cinnamon, baking soda, almond flour, and oat flour.

3. In a different bowl, mix the eggs, coconut oil, honey, sliced apples, and walnuts.

4. Add the wet components to the dry ones and whisk to combine all the ingredients.

5. Line the bottom of a muffin, filling them 2/3 of the way full.

6. In a preheated oven, bake the cake for 18 to 20 minutes.

7. Allow muffins to completely cool before eating.

Nutritional Value: Per serving (1 muffin)

Calories: 145

Fat: 9 g

Protein: 3 g

Carbohydrates: 14 g

Fiber: 1 g

Sugars: 8 g

Savoury Spinach Breakfast Frittata

With this savory spinach breakfast frittata, you are sure to start your day off right.

Ingredients:

- 1 tablespoon olive oil

- 1/4 cup diced onion

- 1/2 cup diced red pepper

- 1/2 cup fresh spinach leaves

- 6 eggs

- 2 tablespoons grated parmesan cheese

- Salt and pepper to taste

Cooking Method:

1. Firstly preheat the olive oil in a large skillet over medium heat.

2. Add fresh onion and red pepper to sauté the vegetables for a number of minutes, or until they are tender.

3. Add the spinach and continue cooking for an additional minute.

4. In another bowl, mash together the eggs, cheese, salt, and pepper.

5. Whisk everything in the skillet after adding the egg mixture.

6. Cook the eggs for eight to ten minutes, or until they are done.

7. Serve immediately.

Nutritional Value: Per serving (1 serving)

Calories: 168

Fat: 12 g

Protein: 11 g

Carbohydrates: 4 g

Fiber: 1 g

Sugars: 1 g

Asparagus and Spinach Quiche

With this delectable quiche with asparagus and spinach, you can start your day off correctly! It's wonderful for a quick breakfast on the go, and you'll love it.

Ingredients:

- 1 tablespoon olive oil

- 1/2 cup diced onion

- 5 asparagus spears, cut into 1-inch pieces

- 1/2 cup fresh spinach leaves

- 4 eggs

- 1/4 cup skim milk

- 1/4 cup grated parmesan cheese

- Salt and pepper to taste

- 2 tablespoons chopped fresh parsley

Cooking Method:

1. Turn the oven's temperature to 350.

2. Preheat the fresh olive oil in a large skillet over medium heat.

3. Asparagus and onion should be added to the pan and cooked for four to five minutes, or until tender.

4. Add the spinach and continue cooking for an additional minute.

5. In another bowl, mix the eggs, milk, cheese, salt, and pepper.

6. Whisk everything in the skillet after adding the egg mixture.

7. Bake it for twenty-five to thirty minutes or until brown.

8. After taking the dish out of the oven, garnish it with chopped parsley.

9. Serve warm.

Nutritional Value: Per serving (1 slice)

Calories: 103

Fat: 6 g

Protein: 8 g

Carbohydrates: 3 g

Fiber: 1 g

Sugars: 1 g

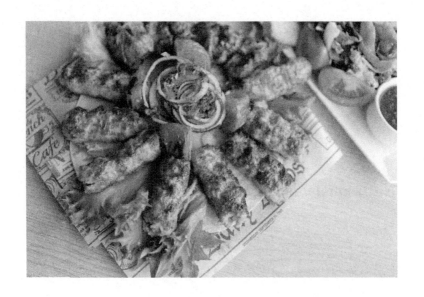

Chapter 7: Lunch

Grilled Turkey and Veggie Kabobs

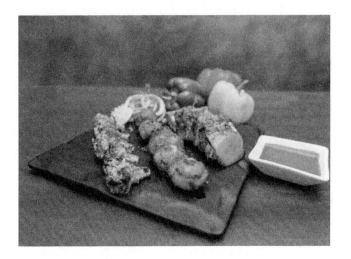

Try these turkey and veggie kabobs for a delightful and nutrient-dense lunch that is also high in protein.

Ingredients:

- 2-3 ounces of roasted, cubed turkey

- 4-5 white button mushrooms

- 1/2 bell pepper, cored and cubed

- 1/2 zucchini, cubed

- 1/2 red onion, cubed

- 2 tablespoons of olive oil

- Pinch of garlic powder

- Pinch of onion powder

- Salt and pepper to taste

Cooking Method:

1. Preheat the grill to medium-high.

2. In a big bowl, combine the turkey, mushrooms, bell pepper, zucchini, and red onion.

3. Toss the potatoes, carrots, and turkey with 2 tablespoons of extra virgin olive oil.

4. Add salt, pepper, onion powder, and garlic powder to everything.

5. Place the skewer of turkey and vegetables on the hot grill.

6. Grill the kabobs for about 18 minutes, flipping them over halfway through.

7. Serve the dish with lemon wedges.

Nutritional Value

This delicious and nutritious kabob is low in sodium and cholesterol and provides plenty of vitamins A and C. It has 12 grams per serving. It also contains 3.2 grams of fat and 3.2 grams of sugar.

Eggplant Lasagna

This eggplant lasagna is a fantastic meat-free choice for people looking to spice up their lunch.

Ingredients:

- 2 eggplants, sliced into ½-inch slices

- 1 tablespoon olive oil

- Salt and pepper to taste

- 1 onion, diced

- 2 cloves garlic, minced

- ½ teaspoon Italian seasoning

- 1 28ounce can of crushed tomatoes

- 2 cups of ricotta cheese

- 2 cups of mozzarella cheese

- ¼ cup Parmesan cheese, grated

Cooking Method:

1. Oven temperature: 375 degrees

The eggplant slices should be arranged on a baking pan and brushed with oil.

3. Include some pepper and salt.

4. The eggplant needs to bake for 15 minutes.

5. Warm-up 2 tablespoons of olive oil in a large skillet.

6. Add the garlic and onions, and cook for about 5 minutes or until fragrant.

7. Add the Italian seasoning and smashed tomatoes, then cook for 5 minutes.

8. In a 9x13-inch baking dish, start by layering sliced eggplant on top. Then put on ricotta cheese and tomato sauce.

9. Repeat layering with the remaining ingredients.

10. Sprinkle some Parmesan and mozzarella cheese on top, then bake for 20 minutes.

Nutritional Value: 21 grams of protein, 19 grams of fat, and 7.8 grams of sugar.

Curry Broccoli Soup

This light yet flavorful soup is sure to be a crowd-pleaser.

Ingredients:

- 2 tablespoons of olive oil

- ½ onion, diced

- 2 cloves of garlic, minced

- 2 tablespoons of curry powder

- ½ teaspoon of garlic powder

- ½ teaspoon of onion powder

- Salt and pepper to taste

- 2 heads of broccoli, chopped

- 4 cups of vegetable broth

- ½ cup of coconut milk

- Squeeze of lemon juice

Cooking Method:

1. Warm-up 2 tablespoons of olive oil in a large saucepan.

2. When the onions and garlic are added, simmer for approximately five minutes, until flavorful.

3. After adding the curry powder, garlic powder, onion powder, salt, and pepper, cook for one minute.

4. Add the broccoli and vegetable broth.

5. Boil the mixture first, then simmer it.

6. Stir occasionally during the 15 minutes of cooking.

Increase the heat to 7 before adding the coconut milk.

8. Reduce the heat, then let the dish simmer for five minutes.

9. Use an immersion blender (or transfer to a blender) to smooth up the soup.

10. Add a little lemon juice.

Nutritional Value: 6.2 grams of fat, 1.4 grams of sugar, and 23.8 grams of protein per serving.

Greek Quinoa Salad

This cool and delicious salad is the perfect meal on a hot summer day.

Ingredients:

- 1 cup quinoa, cooked

- ½ cup cucumber, seeded and diced

- ½ cup grape tomatoes, halved

- ½ cup feta cheese, crumbled

- ½ cup Kalamata olives, halved

- 2 tablespoons olive oil

- 2 teaspoons red wine vinegar

- 1 teaspoon dried oregano

- Juice of ½ lemon

- Salt and pepper to taste

Cooking Method:

1. Mix the cooked quinoa, cucumber, tomatoes, feta cheese, and olives.

2. Mix the olive oil, red wine vinegar, oregano, and lemon juice.

3. Spoon the dressing over the quinoa, then thoroughly stir to blend.

4. Top with salt and pepper and serve cold.

Nutritional Value: This flavorful quinoa salad is a great source of zinc, iron, and Vitamin C. It has 13.4 grams of fat, 2.1 grams of sugar, and 8.9 grams of protein per serving.

Baked Cod with Almond Crumble

The flaky, savory cod dish with almond crumble is simple but delightful.

Ingredients:

- 4 fillets of cod (about 4 ounces each)

- Salt and pepper to taste

- 2 tablespoons of melted butter

- 2 tablespoons of olive oil

- ½ cup of almond flour

- ¼ cup of Parmesan cheese, grated

- 2 tablespoons of butter, melted

- Juice of ½ lemon

Cooking Method:

1. The oven should first be heated to 375 degrees.

2. Cod fillets should be salted and peppered before being put on a baking sheet.

3. Include some melted butter and olive oil.

4. In a separate dish, mix the melted butter, almond flour, Parmesan cheese, salt, and pepper.

5. Sprinkle the crumbled almonds on top of the fish.

6. Bake the fish for 10 to 12 mins.

7. Before serving, add a squeeze of lemon juice.

Nutritional Value: 25.1 grams of fat per serving, 3.6 grams of sugar, and 44.7 grams of protein.

Falafel Wrap

This delicious and filling wrap is made with warm falafel balls and a ton of fresh vegetables.

Ingredients:

- 2 tablespoons of olive oil

- 2 cloves of garlic, minced

- 1 small onion, diced

- 1 can of chickpeas, drained and rinsed

- ¼ cup of cilantro, chopped

- 1 tablespoon of lemon juice

- 1 teaspoon ground cumin

- ½ teaspoon of garlic powder

- ¼ teaspoon of baking soda

- ½ teaspoon of salt

- 2 tablespoons of olive oil

- 4 whole wheat or gluten-free wraps

- ½ cup diced tomatoes

- ½ cup cucumbers, chopped

- ½ cup feta cheese, crumbled

Cooking Method:

1. Warm 2 tablespoons of extra virgin olive oil in a big skillet.

2. Include the onions and garlic, then simmer for about five minutes.

3. Add the baking soda, salt, coriander, cumin, garlic powder, and chickpeas.

4. Cook for 5 minutes, stirring occasionally.

5. Mixt until it is thoroughly combined and the chickpeas are mostly broken down.

6. Scoop out a half cup and roll portions into balls.

7. Cook the falafel balls in a skillet over medium heat for three mins on each side or until golden brown, using 2 tablespoons of olive oil.

8. Place one wrap on a dish and top it with tomatoes, cucumbers, feta cheese, and falafel balls.

9. Plate the wrap after folding it.

Nutritional Value: This flavorful and filling wrap packs plenty of protein with 10 grams per serving. It has 20.6 grams of fat and 5.2 grams of sugar.

Baked Zucchini Fries

The savory and crispy zucchini fries make this meal delicious and healthy.

Ingredients:

- 3 large zucchinis

- 2 tablespoons of olive oil

- 2 tablespoons of almond flour

- ½ teaspoon of garlic powder

- ½ teaspoon of onion powder

- ½ teaspoon of smoked paprika

- Salt and pepper to taste

Cooking Method:

1. Set the oven's temperature to 425°F.

2. Cut the zucchini into slices that are 12 inches thick.

3. Olive oil, smoked paprika, garlic powder, onion powder, salt, pepper, and almond flour should all be combined in a large basin.

4. Toss the zucchini slices into the mixture and stir to evenly coat them.

5. Arrange the zucchini slices on a prepared baking sheet.

6. Bake the fries in the oven for ten minutes, turning them over halfway.

7. Serve with the sauce or dip of your choice.

Nutritional Value: 16.7 grams of fat, 6.2 grams of sugar, and 4 grams of protein.

Lentil and Veggie Stew

This hearty stew is the perfect supper on a chilly winter day.

Ingredients:

- 2 tablespoons of olive oil

- 1 small onion, diced

- 2 cloves of garlic, minced

- 1 teaspoon of smoked paprika

- 1 teaspoon of cumin

- ¼ teaspoon of cayenne pepper

- 2 carrots, diced

- 2 stalks of celery, diced

- 2 cups of vegetable broth

- 1 can of lentils, drained and rinsed

- 2 cups of quartered cremini mushrooms

- 2 tablespoons of tomato paste

- 2 tablespoons of chopped fresh parsley

Cooking Method:

1. Warm 2 tablespoons of extra virgin olive oil in a large pot.

2. When the onions and garlic are added, cook for approximately five minutes, until flavorful.

3. After adding the smoked paprika, cumin, and cayenne pepper, boil the carrots and celery for 5 minutes while stirring occasionally.

4. Add the tomato paste, tomato sauce, lentils, and vegetable broth.

5. Simmer for 10 minutes while stirring often.

6. Add the chopped parsley and continue to simmer for an additional 5 minutes.

7. Serve hot.

Nutritional Value: 12.5 grams of fat, 2.4 grams of sugar, and 16.4 grams of protein per serving.

Chicken Avocado Salad

This delicious salad is the perfect lunch on a sweltering summer day.

Ingredients:

- 4 ounces of cooked chicken, diced

- ½ avocado, diced

- 2 tablespoons of olive oil

- Juice of ½ lemon

- ½ cup cherry tomatoes, halved

- ½ cup cucumber, chopped

- ¼ cup red onion, diced

- 2 tablespoons of crumbled feta

- Salt and pepper to taste

Cooking Method:

1. Mix together the chicken, avocado, cherry tomatoes, cucumber, red onion, feta cheese, olive oil, and lemon juice.

2. Gently whisk each ingredient until they are incorporated.

3. Add pepper and salt to taste.

4. Serve chilled.

Nutritional Value: 17.8 grams of fat, 2.5 grams of sugar, and 16 grams of protein per serving.

Farro Bowl

This flavorful and wholesome farro dish is a great lunch alternative.

Ingredients:

- 2 cups of farro, cooked

- 2 tablespoons of olive oil

- 2 cloves of garlic, minced

- 2 cups of mixed greens, chopped

- 1 cup cherry tomatoes, halved

- ½ cup feta cheese, crumbled

- ½ cup cucumber, chopped

- 2 tablespoons of red wine vinegar

- Salt and pepper to taste

Cooking Method:

1. Warm up two tablespoons of extra virgin olive oil in a big skillet.

2. Stir in the garlic, cooking it for about a minute or until fragrant.

3. Add the mixed greens and cook for 5 minutes or until they are wilted.

4. After turning off the heat, mix in the cooked farro, feta cheese, cucumber, cherry tomatoes, and red wine vinegar.

5. Give everything a good stir before combining.

6. Add pepper and salt to taste.

7. Serve hot.

Nutritional Value: This wholesome and nutritious farro bowl contains 10.9 grams of fat, 2.4 grams of sugar, and 6.4 grams of protein.

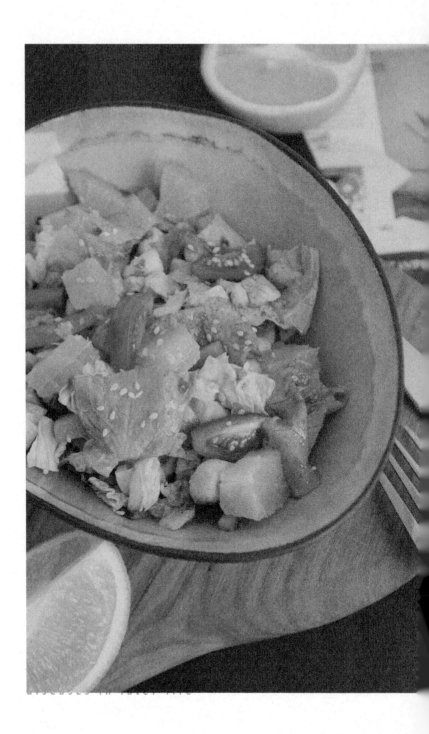

Chapter 8: Dinner

Quick Mediterranean Baked Fish Fillet

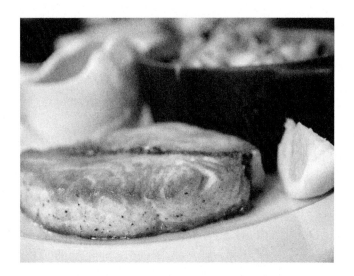

A light and flavorful dish, the Quick Mediterranean Baked Fish Fillet is perfect for those with kidney disease who want to get a nutritious dinner on the table quickly.

Ingredients:

- 2 white fish fillets

- 2 tablespoons olive oil

- 2 teaspoons minced garlic

- 2 tablespoons capers

- 2 tablespoons freshly squeezed lemon juice

- 1 teaspoon dried oregano

- 2 tablespoons freshly chopped parsley

Cooking Methods:

1. Set the oven's temperature to 350°F.

2. Arrange the fish fillets on a lightly greased baking sheet.

3. In a separate bowl, mix the oregano, parsley, oregano oil, capers, lemon juice, and olives.

4. Brush the fish fillets with the mixture.

5. The fish should flake easily after ten to fifteen minutes in the preheated oven.

Nutritional Info:

Calories: 163

Fat: 10g

Sodium: 241mg

Protein: 15g

Lentil and Vegetable Stew

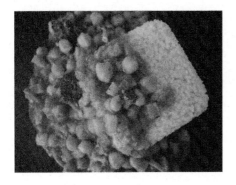

This lentil and vegetable stew is perfect if you're looking for a hearty and cozy supper option for older individuals with kidney disease.

Ingredients:

- 2 tablespoons olive oil

- 1 onion, chopped

- 1 carrot, diced

- 1 celery stalk, diced

- 2 cloves garlic, minced

- 2 cups cooked lentils

- 1 cup vegetable broth

- 1 teaspoon dried thyme

- 1 teaspoon dried oregano

- 1/2 teaspoon ground black pepper

Cooking Methods:

1. First preheat the olive oil in a big pot

2. Add the carrot, onion, and celery by stirring, and simmer for 5 minutes.

3. Add the garlic after one minute of frying.

4. Add the lentils, black pepper, oregano, and vegetable broth.

5. After bringing the mixture to a boil, upon turning down the heat, let it simmer for fifteen minutes.

Nutritional Info:

Calories: 285

Fat: 8g

Sodium: 318mg

Protein: 14g

Sweet Potato Chili

This is the ideal method to take advantage of sweet potatoes' health advantages while still enjoying a tasty and nutritious supper that is ideal for those with renal disease.

Ingredients:

- 1 tablespoon olive oil

- 1 onion, finely chopped

- 2 cloves garlic, minced

- 1 red bell pepper, diced

- 1 green bell pepper, diced

- 1 jalapeño pepper, diced

- 2 cups chopped sweet potatoes

- 2 cups cooked kidney beans

- 1 (14.5 ounce) can of diced tomatoes

- 2 tablespoons chili powder

- 1 teaspoon ground cumin

- 1/2 teaspoon ground black pepper

- 1/2 teaspoon sea salt

Cooking Methods:

1. Begin by warming the olive oil in a big pot over medium heat.

2. Continue cooking for 5 minutes after adding the bell peppers, jalapenos, onion, and garlic.

3. Add sweet potatoes, kidney beans, tomatoes, cumin, chili powder, black pepper, and sea salt.

4. After a brief period of boiling, reduce the heat to a simmer for fifteen minutes.

Nutritional Info:

Calories: 204

Fat: 4g

Sodium: 544mg

Protein: 9g

Cauliflower Rice Stir-Fry

Cauliflower rice stir-fry is a great, healthy, and substantial meal for elderly people with kidney disease.

Ingredients:

- 1 tablespoon olive oil

- 1 onion, diced

- 2 cloves garlic, minced

- 1/2 teaspoon ground ginger

- 2 cups riced cauliflower

- 1 cup frozen mixed vegetables

- 2 tablespoons low-sodium soy sauce

- 2 teaspoons sesame oil

- 2 tablespoons freshly chopped cilantro

Cooking Methods:

1. In a big pan over medium heat, warm the olive oil.

2. Sauté the onion and garlic for 5 minutes after adding them.

3. Prepare the frozen vegetables, ginger, and cauliflower for 5 minutes.

4. Add the soy sauce and sesame oil after another 2 minutes of frying.

5. Add the cilantro and then turn the heat off.

Nutritional Info:

Calories: 141

Fat: 8g

Sodium: 519mg

Protein: 5g

Zucchini Cakes

For people with renal disease, zucchini cakes are a simple and wholesome method to prepare a nutritious dinner.

Ingredients:

- 2 medium zucchini, grated

- 1/2 cup breadcrumbs

- 2 tablespoons freshly grated Parmesan cheese

- 2 large eggs, lightly beaten

- 2 tablespoons chopped fresh parsley

- 1 teaspoon dried oregano

- 1/4 teaspoon sea salt

- 1/4 teaspoon ground black pepper

- 2 tablespoons olive oil

Cooking Methods:

1. Combine the eggs, zucchini, breadcrumbs, Parmesan cheese, parsley, oregano, salt, and pepper.

2. From the mixture, form 12 patties.

3. Heat the fresh olive oil in a large skillet.

4. In batches, cook the patties in the skillet for two to three mins on each side or until golden brown.

Nutritional Info:

Calories: 94

Fat: 5g

Sodium: 209mg

Protein: 6g

Quinoa and Vegetable Enchiladas

An enticing and nutrient-dense dinner option that is great for those with renal disease is quinoa and veggie enchiladas.

Ingredients:

- 2 tablespoons olive oil

- 1 onion, finely chopped

- 1 bell pepper, diced

- 1 jalapeño pepper, diced

- 2 cloves garlic, minced

- 1 cup cooked quinoa

- 1 can of black beans

- 1 (10-ounce) can of mild enchilada sauce

- 1 teaspoon chili powder

- 1/2 teaspoon ground cumin

- 6 whole wheat tortillas

- 2 tablespoons freshly chopped cilantro

Cooking Methods:

1. Set the oven's temperature to 350°F.

2. Preheat the olive oil in a large skillet.

3. Continue to sauté for 5 minutes after adding the garlic, onion, bell pepper, and jalapenos.

4. Add the quinoa, cumin, chili powder, enchilada sauce, and black beans.

5. Stir occasionally while cooking for 5 minutes.

6. Divide the mixture among the tortillas, put them on a lightly greased 9x13 baking dish after rolling them up.

7. Bake for twenty-five to thirty minutes in the preheated oven.

8. Prior to serving, sprinkle the cilantro on top.

Nutritional Info:

Calories: 540

Fat: 14g

Sodium: 578mg

Protein: 16g

Slow Cooker Chicken Spinach Soup

Slow Cooker Chicken Spinach Soup is a warm and healthful soup for persons with renal ailment seeking a filling and delectable dinner.

Ingredients:

- 1 pound boneless, skinless chicken thighs

- 4 cups low-sodium vegetable broth

- 1 onion, chopped

- 2 cloves garlic, minced

- 2 carrots, diced

- 2 celery stalks, diced

- 1 teaspoon dried oregano

- 1 teaspoon dried thyme

- 1 (14.5 ounce) can of diced tomatoes

- 2 cups baby spinach

- 1/4 teaspoon ground black pepper

Cooking Methods:

1. Place the chicken, vegetable broth, onion, garlic, carrots, celery, oregano, and thyme in a slow cooker.

2. Cook on low temp. for 6 to 8 hours.

3. Add the tomatoes, spinach, and black pepper. Cook on high for a further thirty minutes.

4. Serve up and enjoy!

Nutritional Info:

Calories: 281

Fat: 11g

Sodium: 396mg

Protein: 29g

Eggplant Parmesan

If you have renal disease and want to have something savory for dinner, this delectable and healthy recipe is a fantastic option.

Ingredients:

- 2 medium eggplants, sliced

- 2 tablespoons olive oil

- 2 cups low-sodium marinara sauce

- 2 cups freshly grated Parmesan cheese

- 2 tablespoons chopped fresh parsley

Cooking Methods:

1. Set the oven to 350°F.

2. Arrange the cut eggplant on a lightly greased baking sheet.

3. Lightly coat the tops of the eggplant slices with olive oil.

4. Bake the slices in a preheated oven for 10 mins, flipping them over halfway through.

5. Use a buttered 9x13-inch baking dish and marinara sauce to top the eggplant after you remove it from the oven.

6. Bake for Twenty minutes in the heated oven.

7. Before serving, sprinkle the parsley on top.

Nutritional Info:

Calories: 344

Fat: 18g

Sodium 518mg

Protein: 17g

Butternut Squash and White Bean Soup

For a filling and healthy supper option, choose for butternut squash and white bean soup, which is great for those with kidney illness.

Ingredients:

- 2 tablespoons olive oil

- 1 onion, diced

- 2 cloves garlic, minced

- 2 carrots, diced

- 2 teaspoons minced fresh ginger

- 1 butternut squash, peeled and diced

- 4 cups low-sodium vegetable broth

- 2 (14.5 ounce) cans white beans, drained and rinsed

- 2 tablespoons low-sodium soy sauce

- 2 teaspoons apple cider vinegar

- 1 teaspoon ground cumin

- 1/2 teaspoon ground black pepper

Cooking Methods:

1. First warm the olive oil in a big pot over medium heat.

2. Add the carrots, ginger, onion, and garlic and sauté for 5 minutes.

3. Add the butternut squash and bring the vegetable broth to a boil.

4. Reduce the heat and let the meal cook for 10 minutes.

5. Add the white beans, soy sauce, black pepper, cumin, and apple cider vinegar.

6. Continue to cook the butternut squash until it is soft.

7. Puree the ingredients using an immersion blender or a regular blender.

Nutritional Info:

Calories: 243

Fat: 4g

Sodium: 227mg

Protein: 12g

Lentil Stuffed Peppers

Because they are delicious and nutritious, lentil stuffed peppers are the perfect dinner option for seniors with kidney disease.

Ingredients:

- 2 tablespoons olive oil

- 1 onion, diced

- 2 cloves garlic, minced

- 1 teaspoon dried oregano

- 1 teaspoon ground cumin

- 1/2 teaspoon ground coriander

- 1 1/2 cups cooked lentils

- 1 (14.5 ounce) can of diced tomatoes

- 6 bell peppers, halved and seeded

- 2 tablespoons freshly chopped parsley

Cooking Methods:

1. Set the oven to 350°F.

2. In a big skillet, first heat the olive oil.

3. After cooking for five minutes, add the onion and garlic.

4. After adding the oregano, cumin, and coriander, cook for a minute.

5. After adding the lentils and diced tomatoes, simmer for a further 5 minutes.

6. The lentil mixture should be put into the bell pepper halves.

7. Place the peppers in the oven and bake for 25 to 30 minutes. The baking dish should have been lightly greased.

8. Add the parsley as a garnish just before serving.

Nutritional Info:

Calories: 196

Fat: 6g

Sodium: 343mg

Protein: 11g

Chapter 9: Snacks And Desserts

Fig and Walnut Bites

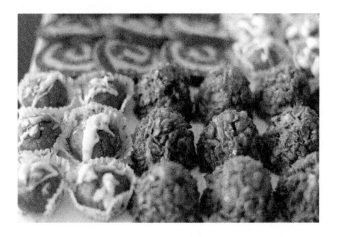

These tasty, bite-sized treats are a great snack for kidney diets. These snacks are full of essential vitamins and minerals, so they won't put an undue strain on your kidneys while satisfying your sweet craving.

Ingredients:

- 6 dried figs, chopped

- 6 dates, chopped

- 1/4 cup of walnuts, chopped

- 2 tablespoons of honey

- 1 tablespoon of cinnamon

- 2 tablespoons of dark chocolate chips

Cooking Method:

1. Set the oven's temperature to 350°F.

2. In a medium bowl, mix the figs, dates, walnuts, honey, and cinnamon.

3. Evenly distribute the mixture onto a prepared baking sheet.

4. Bake for fifteen to eighteen mins in the preheated oven.

5. After the components have cooled, garnish them with chocolate chips. When serving or storing, use an airtight container.

Nutrition Facts (per serving):

Calories: 217, Carbohydrates: 30g, Protein: 3.4g, Fat: 11.4g, Dietary Fiber: 4g, Sodium: 0mg.

Baked Apple Chips

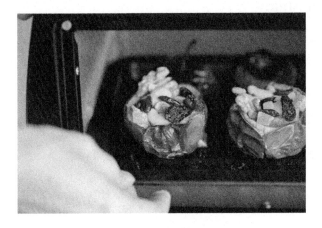

You may treat yourself to a pleasant and nutritious snack by indulging in baked apple chips with a natural sweetness. These chips are great for renal diets since they are extremely rich in adequate fiber and low in sodium.

Ingredients:

- 2 large apples

- 1 teaspoon of cinnamon

- 1 tablespoon of honey

Cooking Method:

1. Start Preheat the oven to 325 degrees Fahrenheit.

2. Using a chef's knife or a mandoline, slice the apples into rings.

3. Use parchment paper to line a baking sheet.

4. Arrange the slices in a single layer on the parchment paper.

5. Drizzle cinnamon and honey over the pieces.

6. Bake for thirty-five to twenty-five minutes.

7. Remove the meal from the oven and let it cool.

Nutrition Facts (per serving):

Calories: 64, Carbohydrates: 16.2g, Protein: 0.2g; fat: 0.2g; dietary fiber: 2.4g; sodium: 0mg.

Zucchini Carrot Fritters

Serve these fritters as a delightful, flavorful snack. Because it has less salt than traditional fried foods, this delicious snack is ideal for kidney diets.

Ingredients:

- 1 zucchini, grated

- 1 carrot, grated

- 2 tablespoons of oats

- 1/4 teaspoon of garlic powder

- 1/4 teaspoon of onion powder

- 3 tablespoons of olive oil

- 1 tablespoon of parsley, finely chopped

Cooking Method:

1. Mix the oats, garlic powder, and onion powder with the grated zucchini and carrot.

2. Heat the olive oil in a sizable nonstick skillet.

3. Divide the batter into four equal portions and shape each into a patty.

4. It is recommended to fry the fritters for three to four mins on each side.

5. Top with the parsley. Serve warm.

Nutrition Facts (per serving):

Calories: 183; carbohydrates: 12.3g; protein: 3.2g; fat: 14.3g; dietary fiber: 2.9g; sodium: 0mg.

Banana Almond Energy Bites

These snacks are healthy and naturally delicious. Given that they are packed with fiber and other essential vitamins and minerals, these bites make a great snack for kidney diets.

Ingredients:

- 1 ripe banana

- 1 cup of rolled oats

- 1/2 cup of almond butter

- 1 teaspoon of cinnamon

- 1 tablespoon of cocoa powder

- 1 tablespoon of honey

Cooking Method:

1. To make it creamy, mash the banana in a medium bowl.

2. Add the rolled oats, honey, cocoa powder, cinnamon, and cocoa.

3. Thoroughly blend everything together.

4. Mold the mixture into balls and set them on a baking sheet.

5. Chill for 15 minutes to firm up.

6. Enjoy or store in an airtight container.

Nutrition Facts (per serving):

Calories: 167; carbohydrates: 18.4g; protein: 4g; fat: 9.2g; dietary fiber: 2.6g; sodium: 2.5mg.

Vegan Chocolate Mousse

Take pleasure in a rich, creamy dessert without worrying about taxing your kidneys. This dessert is a fantastic option for kidney diets because it is loaded with important vitamins and minerals.

Ingredients:

- 2 ripe avocados

- 1/4 cup of almond milk

- 1/3 cup of cocoa powder

- 2 tablespoons of maple syrup

- 1/2 teaspoon of vanilla extract

- Pinch of sea salt

Cooking Method:

1. Place the avocados, almond milk, cocoa sea salt, vanilla bean extract, maple syrup, and powder in a food processor.

2. Blend until creamy and smooth.

3. Ladle the mousse into bowls or serving glasses.

4. Place for at least one hour in the refrigerator.

5. Take pleasure in or keep in an airtight container. er.

Nutrition Facts (per serving):

Calories: 190; carbohydrates: 16.2g; protein: 3.3g; fat: 12.6g; dietary fiber: 6.6g; sodium: 106mg.

Quinoa Fruit Parfait

This parfait is a naturally delicious and wholesome snack. This snack is excellent for kidney diets since it is high in fiber and other necessary vitamins and minerals.

Ingredients:

- 1 cup of cooked quinoa

- 1/2 cup of unsweetened almond milk

- 1/4 cup of sliced almonds

- 1/4 cup of unsweetened shredded coconut

- 1/2 teaspoon of ground cinnamon

- 1/2 cup of diced mango

- 1/2 cup of diced pineapple

Cooking Method:

1. Combine the cooked quinoa, almond milk, almonds, coconut, and cinnamon in a medium bowl.

2. Divide the quinoa mixture across two glasses or bowls.

3. Add diced mango and pineapple on top.

4. Enjoy or store in an airtight container.

Nutrition Facts (per serving):

Calories: 248, Carbohydrates: 28.2g, Protein: 6.4g, Fat: 13.3g, Dietary Fiber: 4.3g, Sodium: 30mg

Cauliflower Pizza Bites

Treat yourself to some delectable pizza bits as a snack. This snack is ideal for kidney diets because it is lower in salt than standard pizza.

Ingredients:

- 1 head of cauliflower

- 1/2 cup of grated Parmesan cheese

- 1 teaspoon of dried oregano

- 1/2 teaspoon of onion powder

- 1/2 teaspoon of garlic powder

- 2 large eggs

- 1/4 cup of marinara sauce

- 1/4 cup of shredded mozzarella cheese

Cooking Method:

1. Turn the oven's temperature up to 400 degrees Fahrenheit.

2. Separate the cauliflower florets and add them to the food processor. Process until it resembles rice in consistency.

3. Combine the cooked cauliflower, Parmesan cheese, oregano, onion powder, garlic powder, and eggs in a medium bowl.

4. Shape the mixture into 1-inch patties and line a baking sheet with parchment paper. In a preheated oven, bake for twenty-five to thirty minutes.

5. Spoon some marinara sauce on top of each patty after it has finished baking.

6. Top the burgers with mozzarella cheese.

7. Bake for a further five to eight minutes to melt the cheese. Use an airtight container for serving or storing.

Nutrition Facts (per serving):

Calories: 170, Carbohydrates: 8.2g, Protein: 12.9g, Fat: 9.9g, Dietary Fiber: 2.8g, Sodium: 250mg.

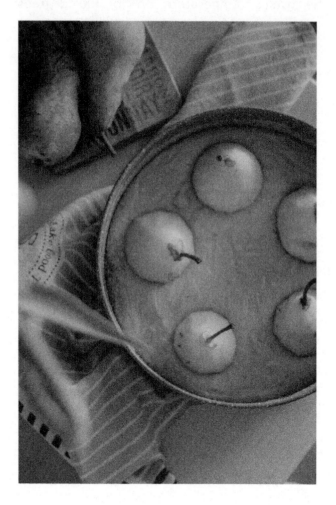

Apple Pancakes

Treat yourself to these apple pancakes for breakfast. This morning classic is perfect for kidney diets since it has less salt than normal pancakes.

Ingredients:

- 1/3 cup of all-purpose flour

- 1/3 cup of rolled oats

- 2 tablespoons of honey

- 1 teaspoon of baking powder

- 1/4 teaspoon of ground cinnamon

- 1/4 teaspoon of ground nutmeg

- 1/2 cup of unsweetened almond milk

- 1 apple, grated

Cooking Method:

1. Whisk together the flour, oats, honey, baking powder, cinnamon, and nutmeg.

2. Include the grated apple and almond milk, and mix to blend.

3. Lightly oil a nonstick skillet and heat it over medium-low heat.

4. Transfer the batter to the skillet in two-tablespoon portions.

5. Cook each side for 1 to 2 minutes.

6. Serve warm with your preferred toppings. Consume immediately or keep in an airtight container.

Nutrition Facts (per serving):

Calories: 185; carbohydrates: 32.2g; protein: 4.8g; fat: 3.3g; dietary fiber: 3.2g; sodium: 170 mg.

Tahini Swirl Brownies

These brownies are a delectable, chocolaty treat. These snacks are simple to incorporate into your kidney diet plan because they contain less sodium than conventional brownies.

Ingredients:

- 1/2 cup of all-purpose flour

- 1/2 teaspoon of baking soda

- 1/4 cup of cocoa powder

- 1/4 teaspoon of ground cinnamon

- 1/4 teaspoon of sea salt

- 2 large eggs

- 1/2 cup of maple syrup

- 1/2 cup of tahini

- 1/4 cup of dark chocolate chips

Cooking Method:

1. Preheat the oven to 350°F.

2. Combine the flour, baking soda, cocoa powder, cinnamon, and salt in a medium bowl.

3. Stir the eggs and maple syrup in a separate basin.

4. Include the tahini and blend.

5. Combine the dry ingredients shortly before adding the liquid components.

6. Place the batter in a greased 8x8-inch baking dish.

7. Scatter the chocolate chips on top and use a knife to stir the tahini.

8. Bake for twenty to twenty-five minutes.

9. Enjoy it or keep it in an airtight jar.

Nutrition Facts (per serving):

Calories: 247; carbohydrates: 27.5g; protein: 5.2g; fat: 14.4g; dietary fiber: 2.8g; sodium: 145 mg.

Poached Pears

These poached pears make a lovely, delectable dessert. This is a fantastic option for kidney diets because it has less sodium than typical sweets.

Ingredients:

- 3 pears, peeled and cored

- 1 teaspoon of grated ginger

- 1/2 teaspoon of ground cinnamon

- 1/2 teaspoon of ground cardamom

- 1/3 cup of honey

- 1/2 cup of unsweetened apple juice

- 1 cup of water

Cooking Method:

1. Combine the ginger, cinnamon, cardamom, honey, apple juice, and water in a medium saucepan. Heat to a moderate simmer while stirring occasionally.

2. Carefully add the pears to the pan, then let them simmer for 10 to 15 minutes.

3. Let the meal cool for ten minutes after turning off the heat.

4. Top with whatever you like.

Nutrition Facts (per serving):

Calories: 124; carbohydrates: 32.7g; protein: 0.6g; fat: 0.2g; dietary fiber: 3.8g; sodium: 3mg.

30-Day Meal plan

DAY 1

Breakfast: Oatmeal, skim milk, blueberries, and almonds (375 calories)

Lunch: Roasted vegetable wrap with hummus and reduced-fat feta cheese (335 calories)

Snack: Applesauce and walnuts (175 calories)

Dinner: Salmon with steamed broccoli and mashed cauliflower (390 calories)

DAY 2

Breakfast: Greek yogurt, banana, and cinnamon (260 calories)

Lunch: Roasted turkey and roasted vegetable salad (330 calories)

Snack: Celery sticks and reduced-fat cream cheese (140 calories)

Dinner: Baked halibut and quinoa with broccoli (335 calories)

DAY 3

Breakfast: Scrambled eggs, spinach, and mushrooms (235 calories)

Lunch: Lentil soup with whole-wheat rolls (320 calories)

Snack: Apple and low-fat cheddar cheese (200 calories)

Dinner: Sautéed shrimp and stir-fried vegetables (355 calories)

DAY 4

Breakfast: Low-fat Greek yogurt with chia seeds and almonds (310 calories)

Lunch: Roasted vegetable and hummus wrap (355 calories)

Snack: Celery sticks and almond butter (175 calories)

Dinner: Grilled chicken with steamed asparagus (290 calories)

DAY 5

Breakfast: A smoothie made with banana, almond milk, and almond butter (320 calories)

Lunch: Broiled salmon with roasted Brussels sprouts (355 calories)

Snack: Carrots and reduced-fat ranch dressing (140 calories)

Dinner: Lentil soup with diced tomatoes and feta cheese (325 calories)

DAY 6

Breakfast: Omelet with mushrooms and onions (275 calories)

Lunch: Grilled turkey sandwich with lettuce and tomatoes (290 calories)

Snack: Applesauce and walnuts (175 calories)

Dinner: Baked sweet potato and steamed spinach (340 calories)

DAY 7

Breakfast: Oatmeal with apples and nuts (340 calories)

Lunch: Roasted turkey and vegetable salad (320 calories)

Snack: Celery sticks and low-fat cottage cheese (150 calories)

Dinner: Grilled chicken with cauliflower mashed potatoes (350 calories)

DAY 8

Breakfast: Almond butter toast and a glass of low-fat milk (270 calories)

Lunch: Hummus and roasted vegetable wrap (325 calories)

Snack: Apple and walnuts (165 calories)

Dinner: Baked salmon with quinoa and roasted tomato (375 calories)

DAY 9

Breakfast: Greek yogurt with banana and walnuts (285 calories)

Lunch: Roasted turkey with roasted carrots (315 calories)

Snack: Celery sticks and reduced-fat cream cheese (140 calories)

Dinner: Sautéed shrimp and stir-fried vegetables (355 calories)

DAY 10

Breakfast: Muffin with peanut butter (310 calories)

Lunch: Minestrone soup with a side of roasted vegetables (340 calories)

Snack: Carrots and reduced-fat ranch dressing (140 calories)

Dinner: Grilled chicken with steamed broccoli (340 calories)

DAY 11

Breakfast: A smoothie made with banana, almond milk, and almond butter (320 calories)

Lunch: Lentil soup with whole-wheat rolls (320 calories)

Snack: Applesauce and walnuts (175 calories)

Dinner: Baked halibut with quinoa and roasted Brussels sprouts (330 calories)

DAY 12

Breakfast: Scrambled eggs, spinach, and mushrooms (235 calories)

Lunch: Roasted turkey sandwich with lettuce and tomatoes (290 calories)

Snack: Apple and low-fat cheddar cheese (200 calories)

Dinner: Salmon with steamed cauliflower and mashed potatoes (375 calories)

DAY 13

Breakfast: Omelet with mushrooms and onions (275 calories)

Lunch: Hummus and roasted vegetable wrap (325 calories)

Snack: Celery sticks and almond butter (175 calories)

Dinner: Baked sweet potato and steamed spinach (340 calories)

DAY 14

Breakfast: Low-fat Greek yogurt with chia seeds and almonds (310 calories)

Lunch: Broiled salmon with roasted Brussels sprouts (355 calories)

Snack: Applesauce and walnuts (175 calories)

Dinner: Grilled chicken with roasted cauliflower (320 calories)

DAY 15

Breakfast: Oatmeal, skim milk, blueberries, and almonds (375 calories)

Lunch: Lentil soup with diced tomatoes and feta cheese (325 calories)

Snack: Celery sticks and low-fat cottage cheese (150 calories)

Dinner: Grilled chicken with steamed asparagus (290 calories)

DAY 16

Breakfast: Almond butter on toast and a glass of low-fat milk (270 calories)

Lunch: Roasted turkey and vegetable salad (320 calories)

Snack: Carrots and Reduced-Fat Ranch dressing (140 calories)

Dinner: Sautéed shrimp and stir-fried vegetables (355 calories)

DAY 17

Breakfast: Muffin with peanut butter (310 calories)

Lunch: Roasted turkey sandwich with lettuce and tomatoes (290 calories)

Snack: Apple and walnuts (165 calories)

Dinner: Baked halibut with quinoa and roasted tomato (375 calories)

DAY 18

Breakfast: Greek yogurt, banana, and cinnamon (260 calories)

Lunch: Minestrone soup with a side of roasted vegetables (340 calories)

Snack: Celery sticks and almond butter (175 calories)

Dinner: Grilled chicken with steamed broccoli (340 calories)

DAY 19

Breakfast: Oatmeal with apples and nuts (340 calories)

Lunch: Hummus and roasted vegetable wrap (325 calories)

Snack: Carrots and reduced-fat ranch dressing (140 calories)

Dinner: Baked salmon with quinoa and roasted vegetable (335 calories)

DAY 20

Breakfast: A smoothie made with banana, almond milk, and almond butter (320 calories)

Lunch: Fontina and grilled vegetable wrap (335 calories)

Snack: Applesauce and walnuts (175 calories)

Dinner: Grilled chicken with cauliflower mashed potatoes (350 calories)

DAY 21

Breakfast: Scrambled eggs, spinach, and mushrooms (235 calories)

Lunch: Lentil soup with whole-wheat rolls (320 calories)

Snack: Celery sticks and reduced-fat cream cheese (140 calories)

Dinner: Salmon with steamed cauliflower and mashed potatoes (390 calories)

DAY 22

Breakfast: Omelet with mushrooms and onions (275 calories)

Lunch: Roasted turkey and vegetable salad (320 calories)

Snack: Apple and low-fat cheddar cheese (200 calories)

Dinner: Baked sweet potato and steamed spinach (340 calories)

DAY 23

Breakfast: Low-fat Greek yogurt with chia seeds and almonds (310 calories)

Lunch: Broiled salmon with roasted Brussels sprouts (355 calories)

Snack: Carrots and reduced-fat ranch dressing (140 calories)

Dinner: Grilled chicken with steamed asparagus (290 calories)

DAY 24

Breakfast: Almond butter toast and a glass of low-fat milk (270 calories)

Lunch: Lentil soup with diced tomatoes and feta cheese (325 calories)

Snack: Celery sticks and almond butter (175 calories)

Dinner: Sautéed shrimp and stir-fried vegetables (355 calories)

DAY 25

Breakfast: Oatmeal, skim milk, blueberries, and almonds (375 calories)

Lunch: Grilled turkey sandwich with lettuce and tomatoes (290 calories)

Snack: Applesauce and walnuts (175 calories)

Dinner: Baked halibut with quinoa and roasted tomato (375 calories)

DAY 26

Breakfast: A smoothie made with banana, almond milk, and almond butter (320 calories)

Lunch: Minestrone soup with a side of roasted vegetables (340 calories)

Snack: Apple and walnuts (165 calories)

Dinner: Grilled chicken with cauliflower mashed potatoes (350 calories)

DAY 27

Breakfast: Muffin with peanut butter (310 calories)

Lunch: Hummus and roasted vegetable wrap (325 calories)

Snack: Celery sticks and reduced-fat cream cheese (140 calories)

Dinner: Baked salmon with quinoa and roasted vegetable (335 calories)

DAY 28

Breakfast: Greek yogurt, banana, and cinnamon (260 calories)

Lunch: Roasted turkey sandwich with lettuce and tomatoes (290 calories)

Snack: Carrots and reduced-fat ranch dressing (140 calories)

Dinner: Grilled chicken with steamed broccoli (340 calories)

DAY 29

Breakfast: Omelet with mushrooms and onions (275 calories)

Lunch: Lentil soup with whole-wheat rolls (320 calories)

Snack: Applesauce and walnuts (175 calories)

Dinner: Salmon with steamed cauliflower and mashed potatoes (390 calories)

DAY 30

Breakfast: Low-fat Greek yogurt with chia seeds and almonds (310 calories)

Lunch: Broiled salmon with roasted Brussels sprouts (355 calories)

Snack: Celery sticks and almond butter (175 calories)

Dinner: Grilled chicken with roasted cauliflower (320 calories)

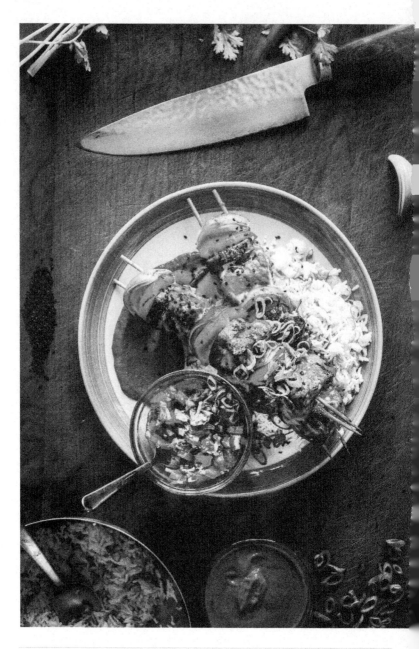

Conclusion

The Kidney Disease Diet Cookbook for Seniors is an excellent resource for elderly individuals suffering from kidney disease. This cookbook provides easy-to-follow recipes utilizing nutrient-rich, low-sodium ingredients that are tailored to the individual's dietary needs. The recipes featured in this cookbook are designed to help seniors manage their kidney disease while still enjoying meals that are flavorful and satisfying. Additionally, the book provides information about the effects of kidney disease on nutrition, as well as important other dietary tips in order to better manage the disease and its symptoms. This book is a valuable resource for seniors who are looking to safely manage their kidney disease through dietary changes.

Printed in Great Britain
by Amazon